I'm Listening

A Guide to Supporting Postpartum Families

2018 Revised Edition

Jane I. Honikman, M.S.

Copyright © 2014 by Jane I. Honikman. All rights reserved.

No part of this publication may be reproduced or transmitted in any form, or by any means, electronic or mechanical, including photocopy, recording, stored in a database, or any information storage, or put into a computer, without the prior written permission from the author.

Disclaimer: The information contained in this publication is advisory only and is not intended to replace sound clinical judgment or individualized patient care. The author disclaims all warranties, whether expressed or implied, including any warranty as the quality, accuracy, safety, or suitability of this information for any particular purpose.

ISBN 978-0692305805

Printed in the United States of America

Cover design and book layout: Dowitcher Designs

To obtain copies of this book, please visit: www.janehonikman.com.

I dedicate this book to the mothers, fathers, and families who have shared their stories with me over the decades. I've learned everything I know from you.

Table of Contents

Forward 7

1. You're Not Alone—I'm Listening 9

    Establishing an Atmosphere of Trust 10

    Spectrum of Postpartum Emotional Reactions 10

    Setting the Stage for Communication 11

    The Universal Message 11

    PPD at a Glance 13

    All Alone in a Crowd 13

    Those at Special Risk for PPD 13

    Frequently Asked Questions and Typical Responses 14

    Universal Needs of all Mothers 15

    The Message of Hope 18

2. The Steps to Wellness 19

    Step One: Education 20

    Step Two: Sleep 22

    Step Three: Nutrition 26

    Step Four: Exercise and Time for Yourself 27

    Step Five: Nonjudgmental Sharing 27

    Step Six: Emotional Support 28

    Step Seven: Practical Support 29

    Step Eight: Referring Callers 29

3. Creating a Plan of Action...33
    Common Reactions to Each of the Steps 34

4. Spirituality and Postpartum Depression 41

5. Broadening Your Horizons—Building a Supportive Community................45
    A Way to Give Back...45
    What the Experts Say..47
    The Next Step...48

Foreword

The following letter—the kind that makes all our efforts seem worthwhile—describes the type of postpartum emotional support I have been offering since I co-founded Postpartum Education for Parents with some friends in 1977:

> *Hello, Jane. In going through my old notes from the period after my daughter was born in March 1998, I came across your name and the great advice you gave me over the phone regarding postpartum depression. Thank you very much for your time then! You gave me the motto, the mantra, and the Steps to Wellness, which I faithfully scribbled down.*
>
> *It was the first time I'd talked to someone in those overwhelming months who understood what I was feeling and helped me to accept that I wasn't to blame. Mine must have been a mild depression, because I began to have better days after a couple of months. I even nursed my daughter until she was 22 months old and I was 4 months pregnant with my son. I avoided all the risk factors I could control when he was born in May 2000, and I never even had the "baby blues."*
>
> *I still have the books you urged me to buy, and I will pass them on when a friend needs them, but until then I've put that period behind me as best I can. You may never realize how much you helped me in that one phone call, but I will always remember your kindness. Thank you again.*
>
> *P.C.*
> *February 2002*

First I wrote My Diary. I did that to share my personal journey that began in 1965. My wakening and experiences as a young woman led me to turn my pain into purpose. I have discovered the need to be open and honest, pragmatic, and helpful. *I'm Listening A Guide to Supporting Postpartum Families* provides a narrative to the thousands of conversations I've had since 1977.

The purpose of this book—the companion to *Community Support for New Families: A Guide to Organizing a Postpartum Parent Support Network in Your Community* (Praeclarus Press, 2013)—is to teach concerned, caring individuals how to help people struggling with pregnancy and/or postpartum depression (PPD) over the phone and by email. In this guide, you'll learn how to respond to all sorts of people: distraught women, upset husbands and partners, anxious relatives, and those just seeking information about PPD.

Chapter 1 "You're Not Alone—I'm Listening" deals with ways of communicating: how to establish trust, set the stage for communication, deliver what I call the Universal Message, and end this part of your conversation on a hopeful note.

Chapter 2 "The Steps to Wellness" presents and discusses the eight Steps to Wellness, which is a tool I developed for empowering individuals and families to help themselves.

Chapter 3 "Creating a Plan of Action" explains how to implement the Steps to help create an individualized plan of action and show them how to assess their strengths and needs.

Chapter 4 "Spirituality and Postpartum Depression" contains my insights on how important spirituality is in the fight against PPD, whether through organized religion or simply having a sense of your life's larger purpose. In addition, there is a wonderful article by a friend of mine on how the faith community can be a powerful force in this battle.

Chapter 5 "Broadening Your Horizons—Building a Supportive Community" is all about how people who have experienced and recovered from PPD can give back to their communities by learning how to help others with this devastating illness.

It is my fondest wish that *I'm Listening—A Guide to Supporting Postpartum Families* will teach its readers to provide quality, personalized support for those battling PPD. We need to keep up the struggle against this illness, which attacks not only women, but also their families—the very heart of human society. Many thanks to those of you who will use this book to become informed, supportive listeners.

Jane I. Honikman
Santa Barbara, Calfiornia
2014

....

Over forty years have passed since my friends and I initiated a radical societal concept. We wanted to support new families in our community. We were feminists and social activists. That meant we believed men and women shared equally in the conception, birthing and raising of our children. We established a postpartum parent support network that has sustained itself since July 1, 1977.

During the 1980s my focus became centered on maternal mental health. I learned about mental health related to childbearing. While the research continues to emphasize the woman I don't believe this is a women's issue. It is time to use the word parent, rather than mother. This edition of *I'm Listening—A Guide to Supporting Postpartum Families* brings men into the equation. I prefer the term "parental mental health."

It is my hope that we will switch our language to be more inclusive. Families and our communities will be healthier if we focus on the mental wellness of all parents.

Jane I. Honikman
Santa Barbara, Calfiornia
July 2018

1. You're Not Alone—I'm Listening

Over the many years I was answering calls to the Postpartum Support International "warmline," I would be asked, "Why are you doing this for me? Are you a doctor or a nurse?" I would answer, "No, I'm a mom and grandmother who understands how you may be feeling. I want to offer you support because no one was there for me when I went through this. I want you to have a better experience."

This is an example of a typical call. In a shaky voice, the woman (we'll call her Tricia) asks if there's a support group near her and then starts to cry. Between sobs, she talks about her fears. Today, before it was even light outside, Tricia had awakened with a sense of doom, a black cloud surrounding her as she gazed at her beautiful two-week-old daughter. She wondered how she could be feeling this way when she wanted to have this baby so badly. She felt anxious, sad, alone, and desperate for help.

Depression and/or anxiety related to childbearing is an under-recognized, under-diagnosed, and under-treated disorder. We now know that at least 10 percent of pregnant and postpartum women suffer from this disorder. Fathers are also affected as well as those who adopt. These individuals need professional help as soon as possible!

This book is about my decades' worth of conversations with postpartum families as a caring support person. My goal here is to encourage others to become involved with helping postpartum families. I'm not a therapist, but a trained, nonjudgmental listener. It's not difficult to offer non-medical, emotional support to distressed people, but it does take time, commitment, and patience.

Tricia is certainly not unique. I know from listening to countless other callers that my first response should be to assure her that I'm there for her—that I want to hear her story. However, first I need to earn her trust. Tricia, like many other new mothers, wants to know if she's going crazy and if she will ever feel like herself again. She shares with me that she didn't feel this way after the births of her other children.

Parents with more than one child can compare their current postpartum experience with previous ones. However, many first-time parents are unsure about whether what they're feeling is actually a postpartum reaction. Tricia tells me that this time it feels different, and her circumstances have changed as well. She describes her sense of isolation from friends and family. Her doctor has offered her medication, but she's nursing and wants more information. She asks me with a note of panic in her voice, "Why is this happening and when will it ever end?"

Tricia and most other people who call for support ask complex questions, and they want quick answers, as well as help finding their way out of the maze of confusion and depression they're experiencing. Many callers are feeling a wide range of emotional reactions to their pregnancy and parenting experiences. My answers are simple and direct; my intention is to reassure, inform, and validate, while not frightening the caller. I can't diagnose an illness or predict an outcome, but I can listen and respond to callers' distress and fear. I care, and—for the moment—I represent their hope for a better tomorrow.

Establishing an Atmosphere of Trust

"Warm," "caring," and "welcoming" are words that describe the tone of voice a listener must have to help a caller. But that's not enough. A caller has to know she can trust you and that you won't make judgments about what she says. My conversation with Tricia, for instance, begins as an open-ended dialogue, a friendly chat.

It's important to learn a few details as you begin a conversation with a caller. You need to know the age of the baby to confirm that the caller is a postpartum parent, and whether this is a first child. Since the term "postpartum" denotes the period from birth through the first year of life, the age of the caller's child focuses the discussion on how long she or he has been experiencing the symptoms she or he describes. The onset of the changes and the intensity and direction of the symptoms will make a difference in your responses to this parent (see below: "Spectrum of Postpartum Emotional Reactions").

If the baby's a newborn or a few months old, I always congratulate the caller and ask about the pregnancy and labor or possibly an adoption. These inquiries reinforce that the status of a new parent, whether it's a first child or not, is extremely relevant. You cannot understate the caller's importance within the circle of their family and as a member of the community. I often remind my callers, as a way of helping them understand how important they are and to boost their self-esteem, that parenthood is unique physically, psychologically, spiritually, and emotionally.

Spectrum of Postpartum Emotional Reactions

"Baby blues:" Crying, irritability, anger, insomnia, exhaustion, tension, anxiety, restlessness

Normal adjustment: Crying/tearfulness, irritability, anger, sleep disturbance, fatigue, dysphoria (sadness), appetite changes, loss of interest in formerly favorite things/activities, anxiety, emotional lability (moodiness), feelings of doubt, postpartum exhaustion (denial of depression/anxiety, feeling overwhelmed, unable to sleep/rest, head or stomach aches)

Postpartum emotional disorders: Postpartum depression (worsening of baby blues or normal adjustment symptoms); postpartum panic (new onset of panic attacks, extreme anxiety, dizziness, shaking, difficulty breathing); postpartum mania (feeling sped up, decreased need for sleep, distractibility, pressured speech, irritability, excitability);

postpartum obsessive-compulsive (repetitive/intrusive thoughts, unwelcome and repulsive/shocking thoughts "out of the blue;") postpartum stress (panic attacks related to trauma, past or current)

Postpartum psychosis: Any symptoms listed above, plus confusion, hallucinations, delusions

—Adapted from *The Postpartum Survival Guide: It Wasn't Supposed to Be Like This*, Anne Dunnewold and Diane Sanford, New Harbinger Publications, 1994.

Setting the Stage for Communication

Before continuing our dialogue, I ask Tricia if she can write down a basic outline of information as we talk (see Chapter 2 for a complete sample outline from a caller's point of view). I say, "Are you alone with the baby now? Can you do this, or is there someone who can take down what we'll discuss or who will watch the children for you?"

It's so important to have the caller jot down a basic outline of our conversation so she can refer to it later and share it with others. Common complaints of postpartum parents are fuzzy thinking and forgetfulness, but using a simple, visual tool such as an outline helps compensate for these temporary problems.

The Universal Message

When I offer postpartum support, my message has a theme. I begin with explaining the concept that I call "**nurturing the parent.**" A motto or mantra that the caller can repeat over and over, it will help the caller take care of him or herself during this difficult period. I ask Tricia to write "mothering the mother" at the top of her paper. It will form a foundation from which she'll eventually develop her own personal plan of action (see Chapter 3).

I believe that if a parent isn't well, the family can't thrive. As I talk with Tricia, I emphasize that she's worthy of receiving care and deserves to be the focus of everyone's attention right now. Unfortunately, our modern view of parenthood has become myopic. We tend to focus on the growth and development of the baby, and forget to look into the eyes and heart of the parent who is responsible for that growing child! Our society is now suffering the inevitable consequences of having such narrow vision: the breakdown of the family, divorce, increased violence, drug and alcohol problems, and a number of other crises.

Tricia responds to the idea of being mothered with a sigh and begins to weep again quietly. She misses not having anyone to look after her, she says. It seems that everyone depends on her now. Tricia says she feels abandoned and overwhelmed, expressing the common feeling that she has completely lost control of her life. She wonders, if no one near her can mother or nurture her, who will? This sounds like a rhetorical question, but she really needs to think about it and come up with her own answer.

I learned about the concept of the need for mothers to be mothered from Dr. Dana Raphael. Dr. Raphael was my first inspiration for helping postpartum families, and later became my mentor. She published *The Tender Gift: Breastfeeding* in 1976, a book that helped me realize that I had not received enough mothering during my own childbearing years. She also introduced the term "doula" to describe a trained person (usually a woman) who supports and assists during labor. There are now postpartum doulas as well, who come into the home of a newborn to help in practical ways such as cleaning, shopping, baby care, and cooking. (Refer to Step 7 Practical Support in Chapter 2.)

It seems obvious that women and men cannot become or be parents alone, and yet the experience of isolation and loneliness among new families is rampant. Couples need to be nurtured in order to recover from pregnancy and childbirth, enabling them, in turn, to nurture their own families.

My **Universal Message** sets callers on the road to regaining control and becoming well and happy again. This message is also what I would say if I only had a minute to speak with someone, since it effectively distills everything I want to communicate into a very brief space. I say to the caller:

Write down three simple sentences:
1. I'm not alone.
2. I'm not to blame for what I'm feeling.
3. I will be well and feel like myself again—this is treatable.

This is a message that parents everywhere should hear. While speaking with Tricia, I pause after each sentence to elicit a comment from her. She starts to cry again when I tell her, "You're not alone even though you feel alone." I've touched the core of her depression, and this time her crying comes as relief. She replies, "You're the first one who understands what I'm feeling and what I've been trying to tell other people. No one else seems to get it."

By telling callers that they're not alone in their suffering, I link each one's experience into our worldwide postpartum network. She's not an outsider, and she's not crazy or unusual. Her cries for help have been heard, and I believe every word she shares. For some, this may be the first validation of their feelings, since until now they've been silent and unaware of the frequency of postpartum depression (PPD). Others may already be educated about PPD and know—intellectually, at least—that many other women and men experience this problem.

 ## PPD at a Glance

"Depression is among the most disabling disorders for women in their childbearing years. For women aged 15–44, it is the leading cause of non-obstetric hospitalization among women in the United States."

—Michael O'Hara. "Postpartum Depression: What We Know." *Journal of Clinical Psychology* 2009.

For more details visit: www.postpartum.net and www.marcesociety.com

All Alone in a Crowd

Some parents have a supportive partner or others who care about them, but they still feel alone emotionally. I explain to such callers that depression is causing that desperate sense of isolation and that there's help for this problem. I reassure them that, having reached out for assistance by calling me or someone similar, they will soon begin noticing improvements in their day-to-day lives.

I ask Tricia what she understood when she wrote down "I'm not to blame for what I'm feeling" (see above, "The Universal Message"). Her answer is one I often hear and reinforces my belief that guilt, shame, and embarrassment are woven into the fabric of the postpartum experience. I find it valuable at this point to repeat that she's not at fault for feeling ill, reminding her that she wouldn't feel guilty over a broken leg or embarrassed to accept help from others while recuperating from the flu.

But psychological distress, let alone mental illness—which still carries a stigma in our society—seems to be especially forbidden for mothers. There's little sympathy for the emotionally distraught parent. Surrounded by the pervasive myth of the perfect parenthood, it's easy to understand why parents blame themselves. In the collision between stigma and myth, mothers and fathers (and thus their families) are the victims.

Those at Special Risk for PPD

Women and men with a family history of depression or anxiety and/or a personal history of emotional difficulties are most at risk for PPD. It's also important to note that anyone who experienced PPD with one child are more likely to suffer it with subsequent births. The ideal community offers a support group or network for this special population. We may not be able to prevent another episode, but preparation and awareness can make a difference.

Current scientific literature indicates that mental illness is linked to a possible genetic vulnerability. I ask each caller if a family has any history of mental illness or alcoholism. Some immediately share what they know. Others quietly ponder, and then slowly discuss the possibilities. In Tricia's case, recalling that her mother has medically treated depression helped her to release the guilt she felt over being ill. I also ask women if they've experienced similar feelings before.

 **Frequently asked questions and typical responses, and ways to steer the conversation:**

What can you do to help me?
I'm available to answer any questions and give you information and referrals.

Is there a support group near me?
Where do you live?

How do I know if I have PPD? Am I still postpartum?
We use the word "postpartum" to describe the first year of your baby's life.

I'm not feeling like myself. I saw a list of symptoms and I have them all.
How old is your baby? (caller answers) *Oh, congratulations!*

Have you told anyone else how you're feeling?

When did you first notice you weren't feeling like yourself?

During my pregnancy... Immediately after delivery... I was okay at first, but at day/week/month it came over me... I'm already taking something my doctor gave me, but it just isn't working... My doctor offered me some medication, but I'm afraid to take anything because I'm nursing...When we adopted our baby...

How long will this last?
The sooner you get help, the sooner you'll feel like yourself again.

Can I call you again?
Yes, anytime, but let me also put you in touch with a support network near you.

Building trust and rapport

- Be an active listener.
- Don't become distracted.
- Restate what you've heard so you understand and the caller knows you've listened.
- Ask the right questions.
- Don't interrogate. Remember to leave time for silence.

- Know the facts.
- Be informative, but don't lecture.
- Convey information only when it's appropriate.
- Never judge, no matter what a caller tells you.

Note: It's helpful for the listener to know how the caller found the telephone number, since it will help your network keep track of how it's reaching people.

Universal Needs of All Parents

There are three universal needs of childbearing women and men, no matter who they are or where they live:

1. A companion or spokesperson through pregnancy, delivery, and the postpartum year
2. Supportive and trained professionals
3. A time and place to share pregnancy, birth, and postpartum experiences

All new families deserve these fundamentals of care and concern, but these needs are frequently unmet. Unfulfilled expectations about being emotionally and physically supported can lead to stress and distress. As a support person listening to these concerns and answering questions, I have an opportunity to fulfill expectations and at least meet the first need. For my callers, I become their temporary companion and friend, albeit a long-distance and anonymous one. As part of the healing process they started with me, they must now find someone with whom they can develop a trusting relationship, such as the baby's extended family; grandparents, a mother substitute, another family member (especially a sibling), or a friend.

Often a woman's midwife or obstetrician fills the second need, at least until the baby's delivered. In the best cases, a new mother receives excellent care both physically and emotionally from this professional even after the baby arrives. This ideal situation is referred to as "continuity of care," and is the key to providing optimum health services. I always ask my callers if they've told their professional caregiver how they're feeling. I also like to find out if that professional has asked the caller how she's doing, and if so, how did the doctor or midwife react to hearing that the patient had symptoms of PPD? Did the person offer her some literature, explain treatment options, or provide contacts for a local support organization? (See Chapter 4 for detailed instructions on referrals.)

After delivery, the pediatrician or family physician may be a parent's main professional contact. The baby is usually the focus of attention, but I want to know if this professional also expresses interest in the parents. Has he or she asked how they are coping? Has the parent been able to discuss her or his concerns openly with the caregiver? The caller's answers reveal a critical component of receiving prompt and appropriate assistance: all professionals must acknowledge that without healthy parents, there can't be a healthy family!

Lastly, a new mother and father must be encouraged to speak about their pregnancy, birth, and postpartum experiences. This simple need is rarely met. In most communities, it's difficult to find an appropriate forum for nonjudgmental listening and sharing. The transition to parenthood can isolate our families from one another. The majority of communities don't offer the type of free, self-help services my friends and I established in Santa Barbara, California in 1977 (Postpartum Education for Parents, www.sbpep.org). However, in most towns and cities there are parent-education programs, crisis intervention teams, and a variety of family-oriented recreational activities.

During my conversations with mothers, fathers and others, I have them start a list of people with whom they might begin to talk openly; family members, work colleagues, faith community members, friends, and/or professionals. Sometimes I remind them that they have to get creative to locate other people who might be going through similar situations. (See Chapter 3: Creating a Plan of Action.)

 **A basic "cheat sheet" for what to expect and how to handle conversations either in person, over the telephone, or through email.**

Types of conversations

- Requests for support
- Requests for information

From whom

- Individuals seeking answers and referrals
- Healthcare and other professionals
- Media
- Potential support volunteers
- Students doing research for school projects

Your goals during the conversation

- Offer emotional comfort, support, and practical suggestions
- Provide accurate information
- Make appropriate referrals

Your voice needs to convey

- Validation
- Reassurance
- Warmth
- Hope

Rules

- All conversations are anonymous
- All conversations are confidential

The Message of Hope

I always end this part of my conversations with callers by repeating what I think of as my "message of hope:" that they will feel good again and that this problem is very treatable. Tricia asks incredulously, "Will I really get better? Is there a real reason why I can't get myself out to do the shopping for fear of a panic attack?" I reassure her and praise her for the courage it took to make this call. Reaching out for assistance is the first step toward her goal of being herself once again. Now that she has shared her story so openly with someone who understands and sympathizes, this woman is on the road to wellness. She has begun to take control of her life.

It's not appropriate to tell anyone with PPD, "Just get outside, go shopping, buy a new dress." Such advice is unhelpful and implies that a simple fix for depression is possible if only a parent "tries harder." Most parents wish that other people, particularly those closest to them, could read their minds. They want their companions, family, friends, and professionals to know intuitively what they need to help them heal, adjust, and cope. Their expectations may not be realistic, but they're common.

How can we meet the needs of childbearing parents and ease the adjustment of our developing families? I believe the answer is simple: all of us who care about children must look into the eyes of their parents, ask questions, express empathy, and offer referrals. We'll discover that the outcome is well worth the effort.

2. The Steps to Wellness

I don't remember when I formulated the "Steps to Wellness" to help postpartum parent callers and their families. I *do* know they work. This systematic approach seems to be an effective way to help women and men who have given birth, miscarried, or adopted and who are encountering problems adjusting to these major life-changes.

I treat calls from partners, husbands, and fathers in the same way. They may be calling or emailing about or for their wife, partner, or baby's mother, with or without her knowledge. In either case, what applies to her also applies to them. The Steps to Wellness work for every member of the family.

Frequently, women who call or write me ask, "Do I have postpartum depression?" and "How can I get better?" I've discovered a clear, concise way to answer these complicated questions. My **Steps to Wellness Outline** also helps the caller determine if she (or he) is, indeed, suffering from a postpartum mood or anxiety disorder. I developed this outline after listening to many lectures by experts, reading professional literature, and remembering what practical, commonsense advice worked for me. It's the kind of advice that I heard from my own mother: "Jane, why don't you take a nap?" "Why aren't you eating better?" "Are you exercising yet?" "Are you getting out of the house?" Those questions used to irritate me. I didn't want to admit it then, but Mom was right. Her nagging was her way of mothering me. I understand now that she was helping me to assess my own situation.

The Steps to Wellness Outline offers information that can be conveyed in a short (ten- to twenty-minute) conversation. (Note: If you're on the phone with a caller longer than that, or in repeated email contact, there's something wrong. It's *not* your job to act as a therapist! The goal is to inform the person and empower her or him to find solutions.) So, after I've made sure there is time to talk (see Chapter 1: "Setting the Stage for Communication") and can take some notes, we start this process together.

There are eight headings on the outline: **1) education, 2) sleep, 3) nutrition, 4) exercise and time for yourself, 5) nonjudgmental sharing, 6) emotional support, 7) practical support, and 8) referrals to resources.** I progress in this specific order, each building on the one before, and listen to the caller's responses. Following the outline gives our conversation direction and purpose. Often I hear a change in a caller's voice as she or he begins to piece together the parts of the situation. She or he sounds calmer and more aware of her or himself. Occasionally there's a giggle as I try to inject a note of humor into a deeply serious subject. Sometimes the caller begins to cry. In either case, the new parent is now on the way to being well again. If the caller is a family member or friend there is also a sense of relief.

Step One: Education

Using Tricia again as our example, I ask her to write down "education" as the first word under the title "Steps to Wellness." I ask if she's read any books, articles, or other information about postpartum depression (PPD), and where she found the Postpartum Support International "warmline" phone number where she's reached me. I ask if she likes to read and if I can suggest a few books on the topic of PPD. Many parents enjoy reading, although their time to do so is short.

Since the first publication of this book there has been a boon to our social support movement and mental health in general. There are many web sites and blogs dedicated to the topic of maternal mental health. Fathers may be mentioned but only briefly. Using the expression parental mental health should improve this situation.

I believe that knowledge is power. Without accurate information, we become passive victims, whereas if we can learn about something, we fear it less. Contrary to the unfortunate and dangerous premise that if a woman finds out about depression and anxiety, she is likely to become depressed and anxious, ignorance is a major barrier to finding appropriate care. This is just as silly as when—back in the "old days"—opponents of educating women about childbirth believed that labor would hurt more if we thought about it. The childbirth education movement and advocates of breastfeeding have also helped by dispelling the myth that women "just know" how to give birth, breastfeed, and care for a newborn without any preparation or education. In addition, there has been a dramatic change in the role of partners with pregnancy, labor, birth, recovery, and parenting in general.

In respect to childbearing, at least, society is beginning to view a mother as a whole being, shifting from the narrow vision of her as merely a vessel that bears, delivers, and nourishes her child to one in which her emotional and intellectual well-being are considered as important factors too. However, men remain on the sidelines.

Classic books on PPD that I recommend:

The New Mother Syndrome: Coping with Postpartum Stress and Depression

Carol Dix's first publication on maternal mental health for the popular press came out in 1985. It's now considered a classic and is out of print, although Amazon.com often carries used copies. Dix is the reason I got into the field of maternal mental health. She gave me my first lessons on the topic beginning in 1984, when she called me during her research for the book. For instance, I learned from her that physicians have studied this area off and on since the time of Hippocrates! Dix decided to write the book when she arrived in the US from England and began having her children. She realized that very few Americans were aware of the potential mental health implications of motherhood—a topic with which many physicians in her homeland were already familiar.

This Isn't What I Expected: Overcoming Postpartum Depression
Karen Kleiman, MSW and Valerie Raskin, MD, 1994

The Postpartum Survival Guide: It Wasn't Supposed to Be Like This
Ann Dunnewold, Ph.D. and Diane Sanford, Ph.D., 1994

Shouldn't I Be Happy? Emotional Problems of Pregnant and Postpartum Women
Shaila Misri, MD, 1995

Overcoming Postpartum Depression and Anxiety
Linda Sebastian, RN, 1998

Just reading or hearing these titles read aloud is therapeutically powerful. They convey comfort and express hope. I used to ask my callers to write them down and repeat them to me, reinforcing that they're not alone because information exists that describes how they've been feeling. Occasionally, I hear a caller mutter, "I *do* want to be happy and this is definitely *not* what I expected," or sometimes one will say, "That's so true—it wasn't supposed to be like this."

I also advise that it's not necessary to read an entire book or "everything" on the internet. Being realistic, I also don't expect a new parent to read any book cover to cover. They will pick out the most salient points. Any one of these four will be more than adequate to answer questions about what is happening to the mother and or father. They all offer explanations and excellent treatment suggestions and practical solutions. In addition, I recommend that she or her supporters call local bookstores and libraries or look online to find what is available. An upset parent shouldn't run around trying to find these resources only to discover that no one is selling them, although this is increasingly unlikely. The Postpartum Support International web site (www.postpartum.net) is an excellent option for information.

There are many other books that contain good information on PPD, but are mostly geared toward adjusting to parenthood.

I call the following books "sequels" to the other "classic" books. They offer insight and wisdom.

When Words Are Not Enough: The Women's Prescription for Depression and Anxiety

Taking antidepressant medication is one of the most difficult treatment decisions for a woman to make, especially when she's nursing a baby. Callers may already have been prescribed an antidepressant but feel ambivalent about this approach to getting better, or they may have been treated previously for a mood disorder. This should not be an easy decision. I believe in being an informed consumer. For those considering taking medication, Raskin's 1997 book addresses this issue. It is important to get the most recent and detailed information on many individual antidepressants and whether they affect nursing.

The Postpartum Husband: Practical Solutions for Living with Postpartum Depression

Karen Kleiman's 2001 book is a discussion of postpartum emotional problems for the woman's partner and other family members and friends. Mood disorders related to childbearing (perinatal) are not "just" a woman's issue. It's a family condition that impacts everyone close to the distressed mother.

Beyond the Blues: Understanding and Treating Prenatal and Postpartum Depression and Anxiety

This 2010 book by Shoshana Bennett, Ph.D. and Pec Indman, Ed.D., MFT is a concise "gem" and one of my all time favorites.

What about Partners?

PPD is not solely a mother's issue. It affects the entire family, but especially partners. I've learned from listening to many callers that partners' primary emotional reaction to PPD is fear. I know what I went through as a mother, but I can only imagine what my husband experienced. Some bewildered, distraught partners ask, "Where did my wife/partner go?" Others wonder, "How can I 'fix' her?" Fortunately, there is a growing awareness about the impact that untreated depression has on "the others," including other children.

Another important concern is having another baby after postpartum depression. Karen Kleiman has addressed this in her 2005 book *What am I thinking?* I cannot place enough emphasis on the importance of open and honest communications for everyone involved.

Step Two: Sleep

This isn't intended to be a funny topic, but hearing "new baby" and "sleep" in the same sentence is almost a joke. First, the pregnancy disrupts a woman's regular sleep cycle, and then the labor and birth upset her inner clock. The next challenge is learning to decipher the infant's needs. During all of these changes, the mother's recovery depends on sleep.

We all need sleep in order to stay healthy and to heal. To repair the body from pregnancy, labor, and delivery takes a certain amount and quality of sleep. Being pregnant and giving birth is a major biological, psychosocial, and emotional experience. In simpler terms, it's a big deal! The complexities of the process fill volumes of textbooks. When I talked to women on the phone, I reminded them to respect these changes and to allow their entire body, from the brain down, to heal through quality sleep. This advice applies to men as well!

The key to healing is *restorative* or *rejuvenating* sleep. The brain is in control and requires a cycle that repeats throughout the night. The pregnant and postpartum woman has difficulty getting deep sleep, when the restorative phase of REM (rapid eye movement) occurs. Her sleep cycle has been interrupted. It feels like a form of torture, because sleep disruption and deprivation are devastating to her body and brain.

It is important to ask the new mother and father if they can sleep *given the opportunity*. I phrase the question this way to get the caller to describe her sensations when she's trying to fall asleep and then when she's trying to stay asleep. For many postpartum women, the brain cannot "shut down" or turn off the thought process no matter how hard they try. Some callers say something like, "I try to take a nap during the day but I can't sleep. My mind is a whirl." Or a woman may relate that she can get to sleep at night but that "once I wake up to feed the baby, I can't get back to sleep. I think over and over about all sorts of things." These descriptions may indicate depression or an anxiety disorder.

As a listener, I take what she has said very seriously and mention that there is help for this situation. I tell her that she should definitely speak with a professional. Perhaps a medical intervention to help her sleep is appropriate. Medication and psychotherapy may be suggested, but the mother and her support network need to learn about depression-related insomnia. I hear so many new parents lament, "If only we could get a good night's sleep, maybe we'd feel better." And of course, they're right.

On a Personal Note

I learned a simple sleep technique from my mother. She told me that when she couldn't get to sleep, she would think of ways to rearrange her kitchen drawers. That may seem strange, but it was her way of "counting sheep," and she swore by it.

I've discovered my own trick for falling asleep: I plan what I'll wear the next day. I pick a color, think about my choices, and then mix and match in my head. In most cases I fall asleep before I can decide on the shoes!

After my daughter was born in 1975, I learned to use a *mantra*—a simple word or phrase repeated over and over to oneself—from the then-popular movement known as Transcendental Meditation. I remember the calm I could induce in myself from that practice. This is another example of our ability to alter the brain's functioning. Somehow these cognitive exercises reach our sleep center in the brain. However, I was also much wiser then than after my son's birth three years earlier. With my second child, my husband and I decided to sleep in the same bed until the baby awoke for her first feeding. After I fed her, she and I stayed together in a bed in her room for the rest of the night. The anxiety I experienced during my second postpartum period was significantly less, both because I didn't have to worry about disturbing my husband and because I didn't have to get in and out of bed all night.

In the first month postpartum, the topic of sleep is extremely important, since psychosis can occur at any point during this period. (It most commonly arises in the third to sixth day after delivery.) This window also varies according to which expert you consult. The topic of postpartum psychosis remains muddled and confused by contradictions and misinformation. However, we do know that it constitutes a loss of contact with reality that is characterized by delusion and hallucinations, and that psychosis can occur even in women with no previous history of mental illness. It's regarded as a medical emergency and requires hospitalization.

 **A Little History Lesson about a Technical Definition of Postpartum Depression**

The 2002 edition of the *Diagnostic and Statistical Manual of Mental Disorder IV, (DSM)* reads: "The specifier with Postpartum Onset can be applied to the current or most recent Major Depressive, Manic, or Mixed Episode of Major Depressive Disorder, Bipolar I Disorder, or Biplor II Disorder or Brief Psychotic Disorder, if onset is within 4 weeks after delivery of a child. In general, the symptomatology of the postpartum Major Depressive, Manic, or Mixed Episode does not differ from the symptomatology in non-postpartum mood episodes and may include psychotic features. A fluctuating course and mood lability may be more common in postpartum episodes. When delusions are present, they often concern the newborn infant (e.g. the newborn is possessed by the devil, has special powers, or is destined for a terrible fate). In both the psychotic and non-psychotic presentations, there may be suicide ideation, obsessional thoughts regarding violence to the child, lack of concentration, and psycho-motor agitation. Women with postpartum Major Depressive Episodes often have severe anxiety, panic attacks, spontaneous crying long after the usual duration of "baby blues" (i.e., 3-7 days postpartum), disinterest in their new infant, and insomnia (more likely to manifest as difficulty falling asleep than as early morning awakening).

Many women feel especially guilty about having depressive feelings at a time when they believe they should be happy. They may be reluctant to discuss their symptoms or their negative feelings toward the child. Less-than-optimal development of the mother-infant relationship may result from the clinical condition itself or from separations from the infant. Infanticide is most often associated with postpartum psychotic episodes that are characterized by command hallucinations to kill the infant or delusions that the infant is possessed, but it can also occur in severe postpartum mood episodes without such specific delusions or hallucinations. Postpartum mood (Major Depressive, Manic, or Mixed) episodes with psychotic features appear to occur in 1 in 500 to 1 in 1000 deliveries and may be more common in primiparous women (first birth). The risk of postpartum episodes with psychotic features is particularly increased for women with prior postpartum mood episodes but is also elevated for those with a prior history of a Mood Disorder (especially Bipolar I Disorder). Once a woman has had a postpartum episode with psychotic features, the risk of recurrence with each subsequent delivery is between 30% and 50%. There is also some evidence of increased risk of postpartum psychotic mood episodes among women without a history of Mood Disorders with a family history of Bipolar Disorders. Postpartum episodes must be differentiated from delirium occurring in the postpartum period which is distinguished by a decreased level of awareness or attention."

—*Diagnostic and Statistical Manual of Mental Disorders IV,* 1994 (most recent as of 2002)

The most recent *DSM–V* (5th edition) was updated and published in 2013. It includes "with peripartum onset" to broaden the scope of mood episodes during pregnancy.

A new mother's partner and support team have to monitor both whether she *can* sleep and if she *is* sleeping. Days without sleep can bring on agitation and other symptoms of mania. A woman in such a condition may be a danger to herself and her baby, and should never be left alone. The woman who becomes severely depressed after delivery of her child often loses the ability to function normally. She may drag herself to attend to the baby's physical needs, but her brain chemistry is unbalanced. Even many hours of sleep are not restorative. Psychiatric evaluation is absolutely necessary in either of these extreme cases.

Harvey Karp, M.D. is a pediatrician and the author of *The Happiest Baby on the Block* and the *Happiest Toddler on the Block*. His 2012 *The Happiest Baby Guide to Great Sleep* includes more good advice for parents.

A Note about Intrusive, Repetitive Thoughts

I learned about a mother's horror of harming her new baby in a PEP distress support group. She told me in private that she had a fear of knives and other sharp objects and had gone so far as to remove all of these from her kitchen drawers. This woman was completely aware of her thoughts and described them as "coming and going without warning." She knew she'd never hurt her baby. Later that year, I attended an international scientific research conference in Scotland. While walking with some colleagues, we shared recent experiences about postpartum women we had helped. One of them, a psychologist, described a mother who had intrusive thoughts and a specific fear of knives! Apparently, such strange thoughts are far from uncommon in the postpartum woman.

These are examples of non-psychotic postpartum reactions. New mothers who experience them need a tremendous amount of reassurance and professional help, even though they're not a danger to their babies. They *know* that they're having absurd, irrational thoughts, whereas a psychotic mother would not. The greatest fear for the mother with PPD or an obsessive-compulsive disorder is that her child will be taken away from her if she tells a professional her thoughts. Sadly, this can and does happen if the professional is not adequately trained. However, an informed professional will know that medication and psychotherapy are effective treatments for this kind of postpartum syndrome.

As I've mentioned, the word "postpartum" is used clinically to indicate the entire year following birth. This implies—correctly, I think—that parents require a full twelve months to recover from the rigors of pregnancy and birth and adjustment to parenting. As a supportive listener, I want to assure a caller that her health is paramount. If she tells me that her next doctor or midwife's appointment is a week or more away and that she's not sleeping well, I strongly urge her to call immediately for assistance. *There's no reason to wait and struggle through another sleepless, miserable night.* Thanks to their increasing awareness of the high incidence of depression and anxiety, many doctors now make an extra effort to squeeze in unexpected appointments with distressed new mothers. Also, it's important to be proactive about PPD—don't wait for the doctor to bring it up.

Step Three: Nutrition

Adequate nutritional intake requires an appetite. That may sound obvious, but it's an often overlooked factor in the health of postpartum women. During pregnancy, a woman's diet and weight gain are primary issues for her. She is weighed at each prenatal visit and this information is recorded in her chart. Her health professionals lecture her about which nutrients her body needs to grow a healthy baby. But what happens after the birth?

"Do you have an appetite?" "When did you last eat?" "What have you eaten today?" "What's there to eat in your kitchen?" These are the kind of questions I ask my callers. Our discussion about eating is similar to the discussion about sleep, since it's common for both of these basic functions to be impaired by PPD and anxiety. One caller might answer, "I'm only eating because I'm breastfeeding, and I have to force myself." Another may admit, "I'm drinking coffee to stay awake." Some women say they literally have no time to eat because of the new demands on them.

While this is no time for a lecture, there's an opportunity here to reiterate that the mother needs to be mothered. I sometimes draw an analogy to the ubiquitous instruction on airliners that says something like, "Put the oxygen mask over your own face before assisting your child." It has to be the same with nutritional intake: first the mother and then the infant. If the mother's not healthy, no one will thrive—including the baby.

Some cultures have rituals and taboos about eating during the postpartum period. For example, in traditional homes in China new mothers are advised to eat a chicken everyday for a month. A family member, usually the mother-in-law, does the cooking and supervises the mother's nutritional intake. This custom may sound silly to some, but the practice reflects a strong belief in mothering the mother.

I believe that many new mothers are chronically malnourished. Often, eating becomes a low priority for them. Many callers complain of having no appetite, usually because of various degrees of depression. To remedy this problem, I suggest "grazing," or eating small amounts on a frequent basis. The idea is to fill the stomach slowly and not let it become empty again. I remind such callers, "You'd never withhold a feeding from your baby, so why are you doing it to yourself?" Nutritional deprivation can become part of a vicious cycle of broken sleep patterns, lack of appetite, and poor nutritional intake. Of course, it's ideal to avoid this downward spiral in the first place, but if there's any sign of it starting, it must be stopped.

In fact, the issue of control is sometimes at work here also. The new mother lost control of her body when she became pregnant, and sometimes her refusal to eat properly after the baby comes is a way of reasserting that control. Perhaps the psychology of negative body image is affecting her thinking. She may be saying to herself, "I'm still fat!" However, I always remind women I see falling into this trap that eating well is part of nurturing themselves. After all, I say, they owe it to their children to give them a healthy mother.

Step Four: Exercise and Time for Yourself

Well-meaning advice givers often admonish new mothers to start exercising, saying it will make them feel better. While this may be true and a good tip, it has to be expressed gently. There are a number of important factors that dictate whether a woman can begin or resume an exercise program after giving birth, such as how long ago she delivered and whether she had a cesarean section.

I have combined "exercise" with "time for yourself" because putting them together prompts the woman to contemplate her self-worth. For example, we all know that a new mother is lucky if she has time to shower and get dressed, much less be organized and motivated enough to exercise. Hearing the phrase "time for yourself" prompts a caller to begin considering her own needs beyond the basics of sleeping and eating.

When I ask a caller whether she has been getting any exercise she may reply, "I try to take the baby out for a walk everyday." This outing may be a major activity for her. She often adds, "I feel so much better after I've done that." An appropriate response as a listener can be, "Have you found anyone to watch the baby so you can take a walk by yourself?" This question may lead to a conversation about a major roadblock in Step Four.

How can a mother exercise if she has no one to baby sit? I remind such callers that if you can sleep well, eat nutritiously, and exercise regularly, you'll generally feel healthy. However, a mother in distress who is already not eating or sleeping well is unlikely to have the time and energy it takes to find quality childcare. This can lead the conversation back to the theme of "mothering the mother" and about the caller's sense of self-worth.

I use my judgment about where the Step Four conversation should go. I listen closely to my caller's comments about exercise and any time she has for herself, but frankly, this is the step I usually discuss for the shortest time.

Step Five: Nonjudgmental Sharing

Step Five is about sharing emotions with appropriate listeners, and applies to both fathers and mothers. I ask callers if they have told anyone else (besides me) about their feelings. Here are some examples of what I often hear from both men and women:

"No one knows. I'm too embarrassed to tell."

"I've tried to describe it, but no one believes me."

"I told my _____ and they try to help me, but they really don't understand what I'm going through."

"He's so supportive, but I still don't feel any better."

"You won't believe what my doctor told me when I finally got up the nerve to share."

"She won't go see a doctor. I'm exhausted from trying to do my best to please her!"

"I'm afraid if I tell them what I'm thinking they'll take my baby away."

"My family and friends are sick of hearing me complain."

"My husband is very encouraging, but he just wants to fix it."

"I can only tell my mother just so much because I worry about upsetting her."

"That's how I got your telephone number. Someone at work saw me crying. She'd felt depressed after her baby was born too, and told me to call you."

"My wife hates me now. I don't understand what I've done wrong!"

"How can I tell anyone the truth when I know I should be happy?"

"We wanted this baby so badly. We went through years of infertility treatments, so how can I say what I'm feeling now?"

New mothers and fathers are taking a risk when they open up and speak from their hearts. The myths surrounding motherhood and fatherhood are so pervasive that parents fear others will judge them harshly when they express their innermost feelings. I try to validate these feelings and then congratulate the callers for reaching out for help. I ask why they might be encountering negative feedback from people they've tried to talk to. Are their listeners uninformed about mood disorders? Perhaps they're not the appropriate people to turn to. I ask the caller who he or she might trust with a discussion of this nature, and to try again to seek help after learning more from me.

I distinctly remember myself as a postpartum mom wishing that my husband could read my mind and just do everything "right." Like pretty much all women, I had formed expectations of my partner prior to becoming a mother. Why didn't he just understand that I was exhausted? Couldn't he see with his own eyes that I needed help? What did he think I did all day long, watch TV? Couldn't he sense that sex was the last thing on my mind? I realize now that I was passing judgment on him without giving him the opportunity to discuss these issues with me.

As new parents, we were trying to manage on our own. In addition to experiencing the usual problems during our adjustment to parenthood, I was also covering up my own emotional turmoil. In doing so, I wasn't doing any of us a favor. It's difficult to learn to speak openly and honestly and be listened to with warmth and compassion.

Step Six: Emotional Support

After discussing Step Five, my callers know that they should be receiving a generous amount of emotional support. However, it's hard to find someone to listen who is willing and able to take the necessary time. Empathy requires caring and a sense of self. If the person with whom a caller tries to share is dealing with his or her own personal problems, that person is unlikely to be able to offer support right now.

New parents usually seek advice and emotional support from people who have "been there." Ideally, such support comes from family members and friends. However, professionals, acquaintances at work, and people in the faith communities are also viable options. There are also phone networks like PEP in Santa Barbara. With the Internet, another source of support is only a few clicks away. There are now blogs, chat rooms, and bulletin boards devoted to providing links between those in need of a good listener and those willing to offer support. It's unfortunate that it sometimes takes a long-distance call or a computer to receive something as essential as emotional support, but we're fortunate to have technology that allows us to extend our search for ways to maintain our emotional health.

Step Seven: Practical Support

I was recently told of a new mother who put this message on her voice mail : "Hi, thanks for calling. Mother and baby are doing well. Please don't ring the doorbell when you stop by, and if you've been kind enough to bring us food, just leave it at the front door. Thanks again!" This example of an assertive request for practical support is rare. Many parents are reluctant or embarrassed to ask for help. There seems to be a vicious rumor circulating these days that it's possible—and even expected—that you can care for yourself, a home, and an infant alone. But, like most malicious gossip, this is false. Women were never intended to mother alone. It takes teamwork to parent! Only in very recent times have humans forgotten the ancient concept of a clan comprising many families that all help each other.

During pregnancy is the ideal time to prepare for the practical side of the postpartum period. The concept of preparation for parenthood is a noble one. Unfortunately, it can only be tested with reality. Every "things to do" list looks good on paper before the baby arrives, but bringing that beautiful newborn into the picture will wipe out even the best-laid plans. Thus, it's worth the effort to talk about options for getting help.

If relatives or friends can't help the new family, then it's an investment in the family's mental health to pay for household assistance, childcare, and/or take-out meals for a while after the baby comes. A new industry has emerged in many developed countries that fills this need, offering professional postpartum care assistants who cook, clean, shop, and, most important, mother the new mother.

Step Eight: Referrals to Professionals and Other Resources

Some of the people who have called me initiated contact with Postpartum Support International because they're looking for a support group or professional in their own community. They ask specifically, "Do you have the name of someone with experience in postpartum depression?"

From my years of experience, I've learned that these callers want more than a quick answer. Almost invariably, they're upset, they're confused, and they need a chance to organize their thoughts by talking with me and having me ask the right questions. I've also learned that it's unethical merely to give out a name without conducting a proper conversation in which I ascertain what's happening with the caller.

My first experience with the growing industry known as "resource and referrals," or R&R, was in the 1980s, when I first became an advocate for quality childcare in my community. One of the rules of R&R is that the caller should receive three names. This maintains the appearance of objectivity and avoids the chance that the referring organization will get in trouble if the caller doesn't like the person whom he or she calls.

There still isn't an extensive resource list of trained professionals and support organizations in the field of maternal mental health, although the numbers are slowly growing. It remains a hit-and-miss process and, in my opinion, is completely inadequate. It's an affront to families everywhere that this situation continues.

Postpartum Support International has a network of support coordinators on their website. Being listed indicates that the professional is involved with maternal mental health in some capacity, but there's no way to ensure a good match.

When a caller has decided that it's time to seek professional help, the conversation can go in several different directions. Following are some examples of questions I often ask before I offer referrals, and why:

Financial

"Is money an issue?"

"Do you have insurance?" (I ask them to look on the referral list from their insurance company, where they will find names divided by profession.)

I explain that professionals are labeled by the initials after their last names. "MD" indicates a medical doctor who can prescribe medications (including psychiatrists); "PhD" indicates a psychologist, who cannot write prescriptions; "NP" indicates a nurse practitioner, who can write prescriptions; "CNM" indicates a certified nurse-midwife and "CNRM" indicates a certified registered nurse-midwife, both of whom can also write prescriptions. There are social agencies in every community that offer counseling on a sliding scale with professionals who have earned an MFT (marriage-family therapist) degree or an LCSW (licensed clinical social worker) certificate.

Medical resources

"Do you have a primary-care doctor?"

If the caller has one, the doctor will likely be able to give a referral to a psychiatrist, if necessary.

If I have referrals to give this caller, I like to mention briefly how they can get the most from their visit with the physician or other health-care provider and how to choose the one that's right for them. I stress that when the caller sees the professional, he or she must put full trust in that person and describe everything that's going on. It will waste valuable time to make the professional drag information out of them! In addition, it's ideal that the person whom the caller chooses really has an interest, experience, or expertise in PPD. However, if the professional has little experience but an interest in learning, and he or she has a good rapport with the caller, this is a match for her.

Next, I tell the caller that there's published research indicating that the two most effective forms of therapy for people suffering from PPD are **cognitive** and **interpersonal.** They're both short-term and task-specific therapies—a combination that seems to get PPD resolved as fast as possible—so they save time and money.

Finally, I always make sure to tell my callers (especially if they seem very ill) that if they can't make arrangements to find and get to a counselor or doctor, they should immediately find someone who can do it for them and even take the caller to the appointment. There's simply no reason to be miserable when help is available if you just ask.

This is a good time to assess how your caller is doing. I ask specifically, "How are you feeling now?" or "How has this made you feel? Do you feel any better?" Does he or she seem calm, focused, and able to use the information you've presented to improve his or her situation? If so, consider wrapping up the conversation (see Chapter 3 on how to end a call and how to handle "call-backs"). If not, let's move ahead to find out how to help your callers create their own plan of action to get better.

 ## Caller Outline—Key Points

"Nurturing the Parent"

1. I'm not alone.

2. I'm not to blame for what I'm feeling.

3. I will be well and feel like myself again—this is treatable."

Steps to Wellness

1. Education

Knowledge is power.

Book resources available at amazon.com.

2. Sleep

Do I have the ability to sleep when I have the chance?

Respect physical and emotional changes.

Allow entire body, from the brain down, to heal through quality sleep.

Restorative or *rejuvenating* sleep is key.

3. Nutrition

First me, then baby.

Try grazing—eat frequently in small amounts.

Baby needs healthy mother!

My brain can't heal if I don't eat well.

4. Exercise and time for myself

I'm worthy of time alone.

Exercise is as important as sleeping and eating.

5. Nonjudgmental sharing

List of people I can talk to openly about my feelings without fear of being judged.

Start reaching out.

I need a time and place to talk, talk, talk.

6. Emotional support

I deserve empathy and a good listener.

Family, friends, colleagues, faith communities, support networks, professionals

7. Practical support

If relatives or friends aren't available, get cleaning help, childcare, and/or take-out meals after baby comes.

8. Referrals to resources

Trust person and tell him/her everything that's going on!

Cognitive and/or interpersonal therapies are best for PPD.

3. Creating a Plan of Action

Once I've been talking with a caller for a little while, I suggest that she or he write at the top of another piece of paper: "My Plan of Action." (This is a separate step from the outline we've just created together.) It's hard enough to write an outline of steps you need to take to get well, but it's quite another challenge to take what you've learned and turn it into a workable personal plan. The information contained in the **Steps to Wellness Outline** (see Chapter 2) is geared toward becoming physically, spiritually, and emotionally balanced. This is a holistic model, meaning that the body and mind—how you feel and act—are intertwined.

Helping someone create a personal plan of action begins with helping the caller acknowledge his or her present state of health. Being in denial or ignorant about a condition such as postpartum depression (PPD) is the greatest barrier to being healthy. At this stage, callers can begin a transition from knowing what might be wrong to designing a plan of action for taking care of themselves. This is a bridge from the cognitive to the practical, transforming knowing into doing.

The top priorities of the action plan will be determined by the duration and intensity of a caller's symptoms. These symptoms—and the degree to which the caller recognizes them—are guides to her next steps.

Remember, anytime a caller discloses thoughts and/or plans of suicide, you should regard it as a medical emergency. This is no time to expect her to make decisions. She *must not* be alone. Ask permission to speak with someone else on her behalf.

If a caller isn't sleeping or eating and hasn't told her doctor about these problems, she must be encouraged and empowered to do this first. Ask the caller if she can make that telephone call herself or if she needs help getting someone else to call for her. If you've earned her trust, she will promise to check in with you on her progress.

If a caller is sleeping and eating but not getting out of the house despite wanting to, this becomes her priority. If there are no friends or family members to care for the baby, her next step is to look up resources online if she has a computer or in a phone book while still on the phone with you. Encourage her to make a list of phone numbers of parent-friendly centers. The local public library is another place to find help.

If a caller is looking for other women with whom she can talk and share her experience, give her telephone numbers from your own postpartum resource list. With luck there may be a thriving support organization near her, or if she is well enough you could talk about how she could approach other mothers with same-age children to start a talk-and-play group.

A caller's reactions to each of the eight Steps to Wellness (refer to Chapter 2) form the basis of her personal plan of action. I'll restate the Steps here:

1. *Education:* What do you already know? What have you read? Do you have access to a computer or public library?
2. *Sleep:* Is your sleep restorative?
3. *Nutrition:* When and what are you eating?
4. *Exercise and time for yourself:* Are you getting either of these?
5. *Nonjudgmental sharing:* Can you talk to someone about how you're feeling?
6. *Emotional support:* Do you have this and from whom?
7. *Practical support:* Do you have any?
8. *Referrals to resources:* Do you need any?

A simple self-scoring method I like for the caller to use is to draw a "sunshine smile" or a "frown face" beside each step to indicate how she's doing in that area. A plus or minus sign next to each item works as well. Either method reveals areas where the caller needs to get help.

Common Caller Reactions to Each of the Steps

1. Education

"I can see now that I've been reading the wrong websites and/or books."

"I didn't learn any of this from my pregnancy books."

"I hate to read."

"When am I supposed to read?"

"I don't like technology."

"I learn from what others tell me."

2. Sleep

"My sleep is sporadic. I'm so overwhelmed even though the baby is sleeping through the night."

"I keep waking up and worrying."

"I have a really hard time getting to sleep."

3. Nutrition

"I have no appetite, but I do try to eat something after I've fed the family."

"I've been making myself eat, but only because I'm breastfeeding."

"I eat all the time."

"I had a bagel for breakfast, but skipped lunch."

4. Exercise and Time for Yourself

"Are you kidding? When am I supposed to exercise?"

"Sometimes I take the baby for a walk."

"I got a babysitter and went to have my hair done."

"My husband and I left the baby with a friend and went on a date!"

5. Nonjudgmental Sharing

"We've just moved into town and I don't know anyone."

"I'm in a support group, but everyone else seems so happy."

"My husband's tired of hearing me talk."

"I've been calling my best friend long-distance."

6. Emotional Support

"I told my mother how I'm feeling and she said she was depressed after I was born."

"My in-laws don't know I'm having trouble."

"My husband is supportive, but he works all day."

"I have to go back to work soon."

7. Practical Support

"We can't afford any help and my family is far away."

"My partner cooks and shops."

"My mother-in-law comes over to help, but she's so bossy and interfering."

8. Referrals to Resources

"I have an appointment with my doctor tomorrow."

"I wonder if I could find someone to talk with who has been through this?"

"Is there a support group?"

# Suggestions for You about Each of the Steps

I strongly believe that the caller—as much as possible—needs to lead the conversation about what she will do next. But she may need prompting. Following are some examples of how you could respond to callers on each point:

1. Education

"I know you probably don't have much time to read, but maybe you and your husband can read out loud together. You won't be reading anything from cover to cover, but areas of concern or interest will be easy to find in any of the books or websites I've suggested."

"You mentioned that your mother had PPD. Does she understand what's happening and how to help you? Maybe show your mom the list of books and ask her if she could read and discuss them with you."

2. Sleep

"Therapies and medications can both help you sleep. There are 'sleep hygiene' hints in books, or you can learn deep-relaxation techniques from a trained therapist. Are you breastfeeding? Your medical professional can prescribe sleep medications. Sometimes antidepressants and/or tranquilizers are necessary to help your body heal." (I always caution the caller to discuss this option with her care provider and I tell her not to take over-the-counter products without consulting a professional.)

"You need to call him or her as soon as we get off the phone. This is an important discussion that you must have!"

3. Nutrition

"Have you ever taken an airplane flight and heard the instructions that you should put your own oxygen mask on first and then help others? This applies to new mothers' nutritional needs, too. You need to see yourself as the 'queen' of your family: queens don't go last or eat the least."

"What exactly are your eating habits? Have you discussed your lack of appetite with your doctor? Remember, not being able to sleep or eat are clues that you're suffering from a chemical imbalance."

4. Exercise and Time for Yourself

"Taking the baby out is excellent. What a great start! Have you considered joining a local recreation center or health club that offers childcare during an exercise class? That would be a perfect way to get a break at the same time you're working out."

"It's true that if you're sleeping, eating, and exercising regularly you'll feel pretty good. Exercise can help the brain's sleep and eating centers, too. Let's look for recreation centers that have childcare."

5. Nonjudgmental Sharing

"Since your in-laws don't know how you're feeling, can I assume you're afraid they'll judge you? Have you shared this fear with your husband? Maybe he can discuss this with his parents when you're ready."

"I understand that you feel isolated from family and friends right now. I know this is difficult, but if you can join any type of center, club, or community, you'll meet new people and make friends. The baby is a great reason to start looking for family-centered events. Every time you begin to build friendships, it increases your chances to share how you're feeling."

"Can you think of someone you could call and tell him or her (family member, friend, professional) how you're truly feeling? Write down those names."

6. Emotional Support

"It's important that your mother has shared her postpartum experience with you. Remember when I had you write down the second sentence in the Universal Message? 'I'm not to blame for what I'm feeling.' We know that depression tends to run in families. It's not uncommon to find it being passed through the maternal line. Has your mom been giving you the emotional support you need?"

"You want to know that when you've shared your feelings with someone, that person will give you emotional support in return. Do you feel that's happening in our conversation?"

"Do you belong to a faith community (temple, church, synagogue, mosque, etc.)? The clergy may be a good source of emotional support" (see Chapter 4: "Spirituality and Postpartum Depression").

7. Practical Support

"Without your family being close by to help with household chores and baby care, it can be especially difficult keeping up with daily routines."

"It's wonderful that you have a supportive partner, but remember that you both have full-time jobs. If you're both overwhelmed by the practical part of parenting, it might be time to think of getting an extra pair of hands as an investment in your physical and mental health. Sometimes we have to reconsider previously held beliefs. Even having a cleaning service once a month can be very helpful."

"Faith communities sometimes have a Caring Committee or Sisterhood that can provide you with links for additional practical help."

8. Referrals to Resources

"This has been a long process. You've worked hard. Looking back over your outline and responses to the Steps, what other resources or referrals might be helpful?" (See Chapter 2 Step Eight for in-depth instructions on making referrals.)

"Have you thought of anything else you want to ask or discuss?"

 The spiritual aspect of emotional health is so often overlooked. During my dealings with clergy members of many religions, I've learned that they believe they're a very underused resource for a family's emotional and practical health. All of them assured me that they do not represent a judgmental or punishing god. They are an important resource for people suffering from depression, since the illness often causes feelings of guilt and fear that their god (if they believe in one) is punishing them for some reason. Further, recent scientific thinking indicates a strong link between prayer and mental and physical well-being. Members of the faith community can be very helpful in this area as well (see Chapter 4).

Ending the Call

After you've helped your caller develop her plan of action, you're ready to start winding up the conversation. In the past I always offered my phone number again in case the caller had more questions or just needed to talk. Before I let her go, though, I made sure she had the number of a person closer to her whom she can call for support—ideally someone in her own city or town. When she contacts that person, I also tell her to say, "So and so told me I could call you," since having an introduction makes it easier to pick up the phone.

It's also very important to briefly summarize the things you've talked about with the caller, and to end your conversation on a hopeful, positive note. I like to jot down brief notes for myself while I'm talking to someone. It helps me sum up at the end, and also makes sure I understand her as we go along. My conversations with callers are usually successful—as yours will be—because I'm really saying only what their own mothers would say. The difference is that I'm anonymous and neutral, so they find it easier to take my advice and listen.

Over the years I'd say about one in 100 people called me back at some point, and they were usually in distress. I handled such calls as I would any other—through compassionate listening, informing, and empowering. I also asked a caller who's suffered a relapse whether anything new in her life has occurred, such as moving, a divorce, or starting her period again. Other important issues are whether she's stopped lactating, if she's resumed her normal sex life, how she's sleeping, whether the baby's healthy and happy, if it might be time to consider starting or modifying an antidepressant prescription, and whether she's talked to her doctor about how she's feeling. Then I end the call with a statement like, "I'd love to hear that you're doing better," which has two purposes: giving her permission to reach out for help again if necessary and encouraging her to make progress in finding solutions to her particular troubles.

A Word about Sex, Love, and Intimacy

Ideally, love has been the foundation of our babies' creation. Sometimes the conception is planned, sometimes not. Sexuality changes dramatically for couples during pregnancy and postpartum. Everything changes hormonally for the woman, but not for the man. This is especially true for lactating mothers. Any breakdown of communication about our desire and levels of need for intimacy and sex can lead to hurt and anger.

PPD interferes with adjusting to a major life change, often leaving sex by the wayside. But before divorcing or getting marital or sex therapy, sufferers and their partners need to focus on treating the PPD. If that has been dealt with and there continues to be difficulties, it's time to seek help from other resources.

On rare occasions I've encountered what I term the "problem caller." These repeat callers aren't looking so much for a way to solve their own problems through developing a plan of action—instead they want me to listen to complaints for which they may not truly want to find solutions. Such callers can grow dependent on you if you let them, so you have to practice a kind of "tough love" when you sense that this situation might be developing.

When dealing with this kind of call, I begin asking pointed questions, such as, "What are you going to do next?" or "What could you do to fix that?" It's important to put the ball back in her court so she realizes that—although I sympathize with and care about her—only she can identify and implement solutions to her problems. Remember, it's not your job to be a therapist.

Listener's Guide to Creating the Plan of Action

- Begin with helping caller acknowledge present state of health.

- Duration and intensity of symptoms determine priorities of action plan. Symptoms—and degree to which caller recognizes them—are guides to next steps.

- Basis for caller's plan of action is her reaction to each of the Steps to Wellness (refer to Chapter 2) as you go through them together. Have her draw "sunshine smile," "frown face," or plus/minus signs beside each step to indicate where she needs help.

- Caller, as much as possible, needs to lead conversation about what she will do next. May need prompting.

4. Spirituality and Postpartum Depression

Spirituality becomes important for many people at major life transitions, such as marriage, birth, and death. For some people, a sense of a higher power at work is with them all their lives. For others, this feeling may emerge over time. By "spirituality," I don't necessarily mean organized religion. It could simply be a desire to relate to a greater purpose or a search for life's meaning. For many people in times of crisis, a need for prayer and contact with a higher being to cope with grief, fear, or a sense of desperation becomes very strong.

Through the many families I've worked with over the years, I've learned just how important spirituality can be for those suffering and recovering from childbearing related depression. Some years ago, one mother said she'd been praying very hard to find peace and a respite from her struggle with what she was feeling. Another said the depression she experienced with her second child prompted her to talk to a priest for the first time in years. While he didn't know how to help her, he did call a crisis center, which in turn referred him to the appropriate assistance for his parishioner. This is also a great example of how members of the faith community can be a link to help.

Hoping to make a connection to such a person in my own community, I spoke to the Clergy Association of Santa Barbara. Through that group, I found Reverend Everett Nielson, who agreed to speak at the 2001 Postpartum Support International conference, for which I wanted to include the topic of spirituality. It was at this conference that I heard his outstanding presentation, which I'd like to share with you. Reverend Nielsen was ordained in the Lutheran Church in 1960 and retired in 1998. I believe that while his references may be dated, his message will never be out-of-date.

> *What is your congregation doing to help new mothers? Millions of women believe childbearing is one of life's most significant events. Yet, for many, it's also an excruciating and depressing experience. One woman told me, "I turn purple when some busybody from church comes up to me, cooing about motherhood. They either don't know or can't remember what it's like to be a feeding machine and diaper dispenser. Not to mention what it's like trying to go to the bathroom." For some new moms, the gloom of postpartum depression hovers nearby.*
>
> *In the past year, the media reported two vivid illustrations of tragedy connected to postpartum depression. Marie Osmond, engaging entertainer, left her family. Andrea Yates, a Texas mother, admitted killing her five children, and sits in jail. They are only two of thousands who knew too little, too late about postpartum depression. Fortunately, Marie Osmond got help, has written a book (Behind the Smile: My Journey Out of Postpartum Depression, Warner Books, 2001), and is now an internationally known spokesperson for*

dealing with this frightening and devastating condition. Andrea Yates, on the other hand, still faces the social consequences of her actions, whatever their cause.

The gospel according to Luke tells the story about a young and unmarried Mary getting a message: "You're going to bear a son."

"How can this be?" she asked.

The Messenger told Mary, "...Nothing will be impossible with God." We can only imagine what the neighbors said. For Mary, and for many women since, single or married, young or old, raising a baby presents an incredible challenge. They deserve more than "ordinary" attention. As God's instruments of compassion, what can congregations do to shine light in the darkness?

When asked to make a short list of places to turn to when she's feeling blue about her new baby, the word "congregations" rarely shows up. How come? Do "the faithful" send unintentional messages of shame and judgment to moms who feel afraid, frustrated, irritable, or a host of other "normal" feelings? Sometimes. More often, benign neglect is the culprit.

Imagine with me two congregations. One is ordinary. The other adds something extra.

"Ordinary Church on the Corner" congratulates Emily, the expectant mom, sends her a "congratulations" card when the baby Hannah is born, and puts a rosebud on the altar the following Sunday. Someone brings her a casserole, and asks when they can all expect to see her and Hannah in church. Plans are made for baptism within the first month or two. That's about it until someone asks the pastor, "Is Emily okay? I haven't seen her in church."

Like Ordinary Church, "Extraordinary Church by the Interstate" keeps in touch. Cards, rose buds, and casseroles show up here, too, but with some significant additions.

Extraordinary Church encourages "planning ahead." So, they offer pre-marriage education, using an excellent resource called PREPARE. (See www.smartmarriages.com.)

A "Mentor Couple," trained and supervised by the pastor, leads the expectant couple in discussing the usual relationship issues like communication, conflict management, and family roles. They explain that "baby blues" are normal, though sometimes can lead to postpartum depression. They role-play what it might be like, and talk about the importance of experienced professionals.

Of course, not all babies are born to married couples, and not everyone attends pre-marriage classes. So, the congregation offers coaching classes, providing information about parenting dynamics, professional resources, and congregational support, to both single and married expectant parents.

Extraordinary Church has no medical or counseling personnel among its members, but they identify a single mother and two married grandmothers whose experience and sensitivity make them natural confidants for new mothers. They stay in close touch during the pregnancy. One of them, Martha, visits our fictitious couple, Peter and Brianna, at the hospital the day baby Jonathan is born.

The "Mommy-Care Threesome" sends along a list of things the church can provide, like a crib, stroller, or car seat. Martha tells them, "We've lined up meals for a week. Longer, if you need them. Let us know if there are some foods you don't like."

After Peter and Brianna bring Jonathan home, Martha brings them a tuna casserole, a bowl of salad greens, and loaf of French bread. She admires the baby, and asks, "What's it like for you to be a new mother?"

"I'm exhausted, but I feel like I'm taking part in something sacred." Before Martha leaves, they pray to thank God for a healthy baby.

One morning a few days later, a volunteer drops off some beef stew, and calls Martha to report Brianna seems quiet and withdrawn. "Normally, she's so enthusiastic and talkative," Martha replies. "I'll check on her."

Martha calls later that day to schedule a visit. Brianna answers the door in an old sweatshirt and shorts, hair tousled, and apologetic about the messy house. It's clear Brianna feels down, and doesn't want to talk much. Finally, she admits, "I felt crummy yesterday, so I clicked on the postpartum web site (www.postpartum.net). I took their survey, and I'm feeling almost everything on the list: angry and anxious, fat and trapped. I want to get back to work where I can talk to adults. Peter thinks we ought to see our doctor."

Encouraged by Martha, Brianna has a thorough exam, which rules out a possible thyroid condition, among other things. The doctor prescribes medication for her anxiety and refers her and her husband to a couples' counselor specializing in parenting.

As part of the follow-up, Martha tells them about groups such as La Leche League, for mothers who are nursing (www.lalecheleague.org), and Postpartum Education for Parents www.sbpep.org) as well as about church resources (www.augsburgfortress.org.) She shares a brochure about nursery care at church functions, and pre-school and child care referrals.

Brianna blossoms after several months, and emerges as a strong and healthy leader in the church's ministry with new mothers. They schedule Jonathan's baptism during a Sunday worship service so the grandparents can share the joy and support present in the "church family." After generous application of water with God's promise, Jonathan is lifted high by the pastor to celebrate his identity as "child of God" and "member of the community of faith."

Because Extraordinary Church prepared in advance, kept in close contact, and referred her to professional resources, Brianna received the help she needed and deserved. Prayers, meals, flowers, equipment, and sacramental rituals all contributed to a healthy result.

Ninety percent of new mothers do not move into postpartum depression. Brianna did. Only about 0.1% of all new mothers develop psychoses. Brianna didn't. Most moms will be fine with basic preparation and care. Left without support, however, drastic things can happen.

New moms need not "turn purple" because of the "baby blues." Living in deep darkness is not inevitable, and no one needs to face life alone. Congregations can make a huge difference—by adding something "extra" to "ordinary" ministry.

Spirituality is an aspect so often missing from our thinking on primarily medical issues like PPD, and it's helpful to be reminded how important it is—especially in such a creative way.

Before you begin working with others, explore your own personal spiritual beliefs to make sure that you can be neutral in terms of religion. It's fine if you feel strongly that there is or isn't a God, but refrain from pushing your views on the caller. In other words, your bias— if you have one—shouldn't influence your relationship with him or her. You may also want to consider developing friendships and links within the faith community, because they're truly our allies and friends in the effort to prevent and heal childbearing-related depression.

5. Broadening Your Horizons—
Building a Supportive Community

"The position of woman in any civilization is an index of the advancement of that civilization; the position of woman is gauged best by the care given her at the birth of her child. Accordingly, the advances and regressions of civilization are nowhere seen more clearly than in the story of childbirth."

—Howard W. Haggard, Devils, Drugs and Doctors: The Story of the Science of Healing, from Medicine-Man to Doctor, 1929.

A Way to Give Back

You may discover after you're well again that you have an urge to get involved with the pregnancy and postpartum education and support movement. Perhaps you feel compelled to give back because you appreciate the information and care you received during your own experience. Or perhaps you didn't get correct, appropriate, or prompt assistance and you want to change the system so this doesn't happen to someone else. Your motivation isn't important, but your intent is critical to furthering the field of parental mental health. It may feel like a passion, a personal mission, or just the right thing to do. I feel a little of each of these, and together these motivations have steadied and sustained my work.

A Little History

The care of postpartum women changed when insurance companies and hospital administrators began shortening new mothers' length of stay in hospitals. When I was born in 1945, my mother stayed at the Palo Alto Hospital for three weeks. When I gave birth in 1972, my stay in Goleta Valley Hospital was three *days*. Now many women are lucky to get two full days of care after delivering their babies, and then they're sent home to make due as best they can. To make matters worse, we also commonly lack social structuring of postpartum events and social recognition of role transitions. There are clearly several large gaps here, and our mental health as a society is at risk.

When my girlfriends and I started Postpartum Education for Parents (PEP) in 1977, we started to fill the gap that existed in Santa Barbara, California for new families. We didn't consciously set out to improve mental health or prevent postpartum depression. No one really talked about those concepts at that time. Without knowing it, our formation of PEP met the criteria that define self-help forms of social support.

Volunteer organizations can play a very important part in the support of new families. One of the main contributions they make is providing social support for the isolated mother. "Get out and make new friends" is a noble suggestion, but it can best be done in a community that offers free, self-help postpartum support. This practice is a simple approach. Peer support not only decreases isolation, it offers an atmosphere of common purpose for learning to cope. As early as 1978, the President's Commission on Mental Health recommended increased links between mental health services and community support networks.

Self-help forms of social support should strive to:

- Address needs of at-risk populations (parents-to-be, new parents)
- Confront social isolation
- Serve as new sources of social support during short-term crises, life transitions
- Promote coping skills and self-esteem
- Provide positive role models
- Display benefits of helping others
- Meet needs of under-served portions of population
- Facilitate referrals to professionals when necessary
- Enhance social ties to serve as buffer to stress
- Help people cope with stress and adversity
- Supplement clinical care through friendship and peer support
- Educate professionals about gaps and problems in service delivery
- Assist in development of needed programming for communities
- Promote social action and funding needs
- Promote new collaboration between self-help and professional communities

—Edward J. Madara, *Prevention in Human Services*, V 7, No. 2, 1990, "Maximizing the Potential for Community Self-Help through Clearing House Approaches."

The postpartum parent support movement includes every one of those components. By supporting postpartum mothers and their partners, we can actually lower the number of women and families who are suffering from the consequences of perinatal mental illness such as postpartum depression (PPD).

What the Experts Say

It's reassuring to know that the research literature from those who study this topic confirm that social support plays an important role in the prevention, early intervention, and treatment of PPD. Here are some examples of writings on this topic from experts in the field:

"Peer support, within the health care context, is the provision of emotional, appraisal, and informational assistance by created social network members who possess experiential knowledge of a specific stressor and similar characteristics as the target population, to address a health-related issue of a potentially or actually stressed focal person."

—Cindy-Lee Dennis, *International Journal of Nursing Studies*, 2003

"The relationship between social support and depression appears to be bidirectional. Lack of social support increases the likelihood of depression, and depression seems to impair people's abilities to make social connections."

—Kathleen Kendall-Tackett, *Depression in New Mothers*, 2005

"Telephone based peer support might be effective in preventing postnatal depression among women at high risk. Women are receptive to receiving telephone based peer support and are satisfied with their experience. Lay people who have experienced a similar health problem or stressor can have a positive effect on psychological wellbeing"

—Cindy-Lee Dennis, *British Medical Journal*, 2009

"Psychosocial interventions to reduce or prevent postpartum depression are becoming increasingly popular, and the evidence supporting their efficacy is growing."

—Ricardo F. Muñoz, *American Psychology*, 2012

What You Can Do

We know from years of scientific research and lay observation that our pregnant and postpartum families need help. It's no longer necessary to conduct a needs assessment in your community to determine this. What we don't know is the availability of appropriate information, education, support, and resources in each community.

The United Nations declared 1994 to be the International Year of the Family, while the World Health Organization made it the Year of the Midwife. To do my part in strengthening the link between childbearing and the future of our families, I developed a simple quiz to determine if a community is sensitive to the mental health needs of its mothers. See how your community does!

 # Community Assessment

During Pregnancy or Preadoption

1. Do midwives and obstetricians assess *all* of their patients for psychosocial factors during pregnancy? If they do, what happens next?
2. Are pregnant women and men informed about mental health-related issues? If so, what happens next?
3. Are pregnant women and expectant fathers who are at risk for mood and anxiety disorders referred to mental health professionals with postpartum training? If so, who pays for them?
4. Are midwives and obstetricians familiar with family support agencies and organizations and their services? If so, do they make referrals?
5. Are there free self-help support groups for pregnant and postpartum families? If not, is anyone going to start one?
6. Are childbirth educators informing families about the need for emotional and physical support after birth? If so, can the families afford these services?

After the Baby Arrives

1. Are hospitals and clinics distributing literature about parental mental health and adjustment issues? Is there a local referral phone number or website for new parents?
2. Do family support agencies offer services for postpartum families? If so, do they include phone and group support for mental health issues?
3. Do pediatricians and family physicians assess psychosocial and support needs for the first year postpartum? If so, what happens next?
4. Are new families encouraged to seek support for any and all mental health issues?

If so, congratulations—you live in a beautiful community!

The Next Step

In 2000, I published *Step by Step: A Guide to Organizing a Postpartum Parent Support Network in Your Community,* a workbook that encourages individuals to work as a team to support parents and their families. In 2013 it was updated with a new title, *Community Support for New Families* (available on amazon.com). It provides a guideline or framework that can easily be adapted to achieve the kind of community described in my community assessment.

Establishing a support group and/or network is a very individual experience with no rigid and absolute recipe. There is a process to follow, however, and I'll tell you what it takes to accomplish: time, patience, and commitment. (Remember, these are the same qualities that I mentioned in Chapter 1 as traits of a good volunteer!) My process includes specific steps within six stages. While the steps will vary from community to community, you must pass through each of the six stages to ensure the successful development of a postpartum support network for your community.

These stages are:

- Stage 1 Brainstorming: visualize and start organizing for the parent-support network you would like to create.
- Stage 2 Investigation: research other parent-support groups and networks in your community and beyond
- Stage 3 Planning: formulate and make decisions
- Stage 4 Implementation: new network on its way
- Stage 5 Evaluation: critical process that is often neglected
- Stage 6 Future Endeavors: thinking ahead, new goals to keep the network fresh

I doubt if there's a village in the entire world that's as wonderful as I would like to imagine, but I have a fantasy that somewhere they support postpartum families completely. As we strive toward improving our own villages, towns, and cities, there will be challenges in meeting the needs of every mother, father, and their family. We need to work together now to evaluate and improve current policies and systems of practice for our families surrounding the transition to parenthood.

I know from my personal journey since the 1970s, that we're becoming more sensitive to the mental health needs of families. With the continued expansion of our social support movement—and your help—someday every community will offer pregnancy and postpartum parent support.

Made in the USA
Middletown, DE
01 June 2019